I0413010

The Hope Project

How to inspire your mind, build a business and fight off depression and anxiety.

David Small

THE HOPE PROJECT

Copyright © 2012 David Small

Rev. date: 04-July-2015

Written by: David Small

Edited by: Elizabeth Ridley

David Small's books can be ordered through
www.wanderingleader.com

ISBN: 1507799217
ISBN-13: 978-1507799215

DEDICATION

For TSN's Michael Landsberg. Your documentary
"Darkness and Hope" gave me a voice.

CONTENTS

ACKNOWLEDGMENTS

Thank you to my family and friends. I would have never had the courage to write this book if I didn't know you supported me. Thank you to my editor for helping me be a better writer. Thank you for those of you who support Me+, my life has been changed because of you and I am eternally grateful.

UPDATED VERSION

I published this book originally in January 2012, and then left the next day on a ten day trip to Germany where I wouldn't have any internet access. When I got home I remember the book had been released so I went onto Amazon to check to see how it was doing. I was shocked. The book was #1 in it's category. I clicked refresh a few times to see if my computer just wasn't loading the complete number, but each time the page reloaded, it came up as #1.

This tiny little book has touched many people's lives. I have been so blessed by the emails I've received from people who have read this book. I was moved to tears by an email I received one afternoon from a woman who had just been given a copy of The Hope Project. She started by thanking me for writing it, and then went on to tell me that she had recently lost her husband to suicide. He struggled with depression for years, he hid it, fought it, tried to beat it, and in the end lost the fight. She said she was crying as she read my book because she wished it had gotten into her husbands hands before it was too late. I was so humbled to hear her story, and the stories of so many others who have come face to face with the monster of depression.

Three years since publishing this book I am updating some of the content, refreshing some of the stories, and more so just taking an opportunity to say thank you, to you, my readers, my friends, and the people who support Small World Health. You're not alone in your struggle, there is hope out there.

INTRODUCTION

Writing about depression is, well, a rather depressing topic. I'd much rather just be happy, healthy and wealthy and not need to tell my story. Just like I'd rather that you were happy, healthy and wealthy. But life's just not fair I guess. With feelings of nervousness, like someone standing up at their first AA meeting, I'd stand and say to you, "Hi my name is Dave and I suffer from depression."

They say that no man is an island - and for a lot of my life, and even still sometimes today, I fought against that idea. I thought that I could be self-sufficient, and that I wouldn't need to rely on anyone else for anything. This is all fine and great when the sun is shining. But when a hurricane blows in, and you're all alone on that island you've created, it can be really lonely.

Speaking of islands, one of my dreams in life is to build a little house on an island that my family owns. In the back of the island is a big field, right now it's wild and overgrown. But I can picture it being burned down and cleaned up. I'd build a little cabin on one side of the field, and then plant some rows of grapes on the other side. At the beginning of each row of grapes I'll plant a rose bush. During the summers I'll live out on the island, tending to my grapes, and being at peace with the world. In the fall I'll harvest my grapes and make extraordinary red wine that will inspire my writing all winter. But, I'm sure that when those big storms blow in, there will be times I'll wish I wasn't alone on that island.

I've faced a few (metaphorical) hurricanes in my life, some that I wasn't sure how I was going to get through. Despite my desire to keep all my feelings hidden inside me, sheltered from the world, I'm going to try my best to share them with you now. I don't like talking about my struggles with depression because I feel like I'm exposing a weakness. What if I want to be the Prime Minister[1] one day, and someone pulls out this book and uses my story to say I'm not a good leader. What if someone laughs at my story? And worse yet, what if I'm alone with these feelings and no one can relate to my experiences, or cares...

I'm going to suck it up and despite the fears, share my story with you. I found how I cope with my illness, and I found hope. I found a project that I can hold onto that helped me dream again. I want to share some ideas and methods with you that might help you cope. I want to share my projects with you so I can explain how these things give me hope - and I want to encourage you to start your own Hope Project. These projects will inspire your mind and will help you fight off feelings of depression and anxiety. In my life I've been very blessed. I've coached professional athletes all over the world, I've had books published, and I've started and run businesses. But my goal with this little book is to tell you that you're not alone, to shed some light on this illness, and to offer you some encouragement and stepping-stones to start your own Hope Project.

In my book *The Wandering Leader* (2014) I

---

[1] I'm Canadian

briefly touch on my struggle with depression in one chapter. But I wanted to write a more detailed account of my story. I wanted to get my story into the hands of as many people who might share my struggles. It has nothing to do with me, but it has to do with you. I want you to be encouraged that other people feel the same way, and that other people are there for you.

The sunset at the end of a big storm always gives you a little bit of hope. I want this book to be a lifeline for you - I'm offering you an outstretched hand, take it and come on a journey with me. After all, we're fighting a common war, so we need to support each other.

1. HOT TUB TALKS

I have a good friend who lives on an island. Literally. It's a big island - a couple miles wide - and he lives there year round. In the summer months they boat back and forth to the town (rain or shine). In the winter, the lake freezes and the island residents make an "ice road" and for a short period of time can drive their cars back and forth from the island to town. The toughest months are in the freeze-up and the thaw. When the ice isn't thick enough to drive a vehicle on, but the water isn't open to boat across. During these months the island residents put a small footbridge across the shortest point to the mainland and have to walk. My friend's house is on a beautiful point that looks across a bay into the heart of the small town we grew up in. He has a hot tub on his deck, and there are many nights that we'll light some tiki torches, put on some music, and drink some vodka-OJs while sitting in the hot tub. It's a beautiful place, to enjoy the warm water and look out onto the lights of the city. It's one of the most calm and peaceful places I know in the town. There have been many times that we've sat there talking, sharing stories, until the sun came up the next morning. My friend is a great guy, but he does not understand depression.

As something that I've struggled with in my life, it's come up in a few of our hot tub talks. I've tried to explain it to him many times but as someone who doesn't suffer from depression it's tough for him to wrap his head around it. For him, if something is making him sad, he addresses it and moves on. He doesn't get sad for no reason - and for him that's tough to understand. It's not a lack of compassion or a lack of faith, it's just that it's tough to comprehend something that he can control so well.

If I break my arm and the doctor puts a cast on my arm, my friend can see that and understand that. Something is broken. If I am chopping vegetables and I cut my finger, the doctor may give me some stitches, my friend can see that and understand that. Something is cut. If I am playing soccer and I twist my ankle, it may swell up, my friend can see that. Something is swollen and hurt. But if it's a beautiful day, with birds singing and blue skies and I say "I'm struggling with depression today" - there is nothing to see, and for him and many others, it's tough to understand. Although for us, it feels like something is broken, hurt, and that our hearts are swollen, there is nothing more that we can offer to someone to illustrate this illness. It just takes faith that it's happening, that it's real, and that it's there.

I was diagnosed with depression when I was in my early 20's. I'm sure if we were more publicly educated about the illness I would have been diagnosed years before - but it is still a bit of a "hush hush" topic for many people. Before I can explain what a Hope Project is, I need to first explain how depression has unfolded for me. For me there have been two version of depression - one being situational depression, and the other being biological depression.

First the situational depression. To define this I will say that it's a form of sadness, depression, or anxiety that is brought on by a particular situation. Maybe it's a break up. A firing. An argument. It can really be anything. Some sort of situation triggers something inside me that sends me into a tailspin downwards. Other times it can be because of a lack of sleep. eating poorly or drinking too much. The triggers change as time goes on, they can be good things or bad things, but once something triggers my depression the rest of the day is a write-off.

The second, and for me the more common, is the biological depression. I try to explain this kind of struggle to my friends without depression as a way for them to understand, but it's still hard sometimes. Biological depression is what the doctors' test for. To put it simply, our body produces certain chemicals and hormones. These hormones do everything from regulate energy, sleep, mood, happiness, and countless other things. For me, my body doesn't produce the same amount of the "happiness" hormone (serotonin) that other people might produce. I can't will myself to produce more of the chemical, and unfortunately it's not true that if I "just eat more broccoli" I'll be okay. These missing hormones can't totally be replaced by my diet. So when my body doesn't produce these hormones, it affects my mood. There are lots of pharmaceutical drugs and anti-depressants (SSRIs) out there that artificially produce the hormones for you, or help the hormones move, but we'll get more into that later.

For much of my life - even since I was young - I have been in a leadership role. From being the one to organize and plan the back-yard hockey games on a frozen pond, to coaching elite athletes, or being an officer in the army, to now-a-days owning my own international company and being responsible for employees. Through all of these moments where people are looking to me for answers, my "mood" cannot affect my leadership. For me there was a period of time where I felt that maybe I couldn't be a leader anymore because of this illness. That depression made me "weak" and weakness is a quality that a leader can't have.

2. TRANSITIONS

It started with alcohol. Liquid confidence. Dutch courage some call it. The courage found at the bottom of a bottle. Alcohol is also a nervous system depressant. I'm not a big drinker, I enjoy a social drink with my friends, but overall I'm not a big drinker. In my early 20s when I was at parties I started to notice a pattern. I'd start off the evening having fun and being really happy, but the more I drank, the harder it became to control how I felt. I could tell that it wasn't the alcohol that was making me lose control of my feelings. It may have been helping, but it wasn't the alcohol. The alcohol was just acting as a rollercoaster car - starting with a slow gradual up, followed by a fast wild down. I knew that the feelings I was experiencing were things that I felt when I was sober, but the alcohol was magnifying it. All it seemed I could do was try to hold on for the ride.

I decided to go and speak to a counselor. At the time, I was working in a small city for a sports team. I was the director of operations for the team and the assistant coach. The role was a high profile one, and most people in the city knew who I was. I was in a role that required me to be a leader. As the director of operations I was responsible to lead the direction of the club, the relations with the city, and the recruitment of future players. As a coach I was responsible for leading the athletes. I don't know if I'd have gone to see the counselor if it wasn't for one player. This player was dealing with an alcoholic mother and it was affecting his life and his performance as a player. The team offered to pay for him to go and speak to a counselor about it. He shared with me a lot of the things that he spoke about with the counselor and he shared with me how it was helping him cope. His openness to talk about it and to admit he was going to a counselor encouraged me that it was okay to go. He wasn't ashamed of it. So quietly, I made an appointment.

I have mixed feelings about counselors. I believe that there isn't a single person who couldn't benefit from going to speak to a counselor at some point in their life. Everyone needs an unbiased professional to bounce things off from time to time. In my life I've been to a handful of different counselors and as a businessperson I am always critical of other businesses. I am constantly analyzing people, environments, and businesses. Trying to see what they do well, what could be better, and what is their business model. A counselor's office is no different. I think there are a lot of great counselors out there, who do a good job being professional and caring. But I also think there are a lot of really crappy counselors out there. Counselors who charge too much, care too little, and leave you feel like you're talking to a brick wall. I once spoke to a counselor who charged $175/hour. He had those "transition lenses" in his glasses that would automatically adjust from sunglasses to regular glasses depending on the light in the room. His office was on a corner of a building, with huge windows on all sides that let in a lot of light, thus causing his glasses to be in the "sunglasses" mode for most of the conversation. Imagine sitting there trying to feel comfortable paying $175 to some dork wearing sunglasses. I'd leave those session feeling more pissed off than when I went in.

After a few months speaking with a fairly good counselor, I realized that the "coping methods" weren't really working for me. All I wanted was to be able to control my emotions. I decided to go and speak to our team doctor. The Doc ran some tests on me, and after a couple weeks we met again to talk about the results. He explained to me about the hormones in the body, and that based on the results of the test my body wasn't producing certain hormones. He explained how that would make me feel like I can't control my emotions at times. He explained that it wasn't a severe lack of hormones, but it was enough that I would notice it. As doctors do, he recommended that I start on an anti-depressant called a Selective Serotonin Reuptake Inhibitor (SSRI). Being one who doesn't like taking pills, he tried to comfort me by saying "this is a really popular one. Even my daughter takes this one." I weighed my dislike of medications against how much I wanted to be able to control my feelings and I decided to try out the anti-depressants. I didn't tell anyone.

My personal opinion is that whenever possible it's best not to be on any medications. My chiropractor used to explain it to me like this; if your house was on fire, and your smoke alarm went off in the middle of the night, waking you up, would you go and take the batteries out of the smoke alarm so you can go back to sleep? He explained that taking drugs was just taking the batteries out of the smoke alarm. It isn't addressing the real problem. Now I'm not naive enough to say to never take medications. There is a time and a place that it is important. I just think that whenever possible we should try to address the real problem, or if we can find a natural supplement that works take it in place. If I've got a headache I can either choose to take a pain killer, or I can drink more water and my headache will usually go away. But it's a bit different when I've got a *heartache*. For me, my depression wasn't a severe case, but for some, being on doctor prescribed meds is really important.

There is a quote that says, "The best revenge is living well." I felt like I needed to seek revenge against this illness that was screwing with my life and career - and for me I was going to live as best I could, in hopes to get off the meds and "conquer" the illness. Sadly, it doesn't always work that way.

3. THE FLY

When I was 26 years old, I was laid off from my job of four years. It was a major life-changing event for me. It was difficult and there were lots of tears, but deep down inside I knew that it would become one of the best things for me. I had felt like my career was heading in the right direction. I was networking, making connections with influential people and they seemed to like me. Within a few short years I went from being a relatively unknown coach in Canada to winning a championship, working for two NHL hockey clubs, and being named Director of Operations

for Team Canada Junior A Challenge. I was
working about 60 hours a week, my life was my
job, and through all the best days and all the
worst days, I was taking these anti-depressants. I
was taking these pills during the highest points,
getting to work with Team Canada, one of the
greatest honors of my life, and through the low
points of getting called in and being told I was
being laid off. I just wanted to be in control of my
feelings, good or bad.

After losing my job I moved across the country
back to my hometown. I was embarrassed to be
back home. I felt like I had let everyone down
and I knew that the only thing that would save
me is if I threw myself into another adventure
right away. I hadn't lived in my hometown for
nearly a decade and I wasn't ready to be back
there yet.

Within 30 days of losing my job I was on a plane
to London England where I would try to start a
new life. Within seven weeks of landing in
London I was offered a job working for Apple. I
began a new life in London, one that didn't
involve the pressures of the sports world. The
friends that I made in London didn't care about
me because of my career or job title; they cared
about me because of who I was. It was

refreshing. I began to see a counselor in London. He was one of the better counselors that I've been too and he helped me work through this rocky transition in my life. I had a lot of anger, sadness, and hurt in me from being laid off and he helped me come to grips with it and release it. Slowly I began to wean myself off the anti-depressants.

After eight months living in London, I return to Canada for my brother's wedding. I felt great. I was off the anti-depressants, I had started studying Kung Fu, I had made some amazing friends in London, and most importantly I had regained my confidence as a leader, a coach, and as a person. I felt like I was ready to take on anything.

There is a great little book called *Me²* (Me Squared). The book talks about taking a "quantum leap" in your career. The author explains that sometimes small steps isn't going to get you to the top, rather, taking a quantum leap will help you take the next big step in your career. At the beginning of the book the author illustrates a story that I really like. He's watching a fly buzzing against the window in his house. Across the other side of the room the door is open to outside. This fly is buzzing and buzzing pressing against the glass, trying to get to the freedom of outside, but if he would just turn around and fly the other way for a little while then he'd be free. For a long time I was that fly. I was buzzing around against the glass, trying so hard to break free of the 60-hour workweek and "become someone". It turns out that all I needed to do is turn around and go a different direction for a while and then something will present itself to me.

Since I was little I had the spirit of adventure instilled in me by my family. We travelled all over the world. By age twenty-eight I had been a resident in six different countries. As a sports coach, one thing I'd always wanted to do was to work as a professional head coach in Europe. It was a nice lifestyle, good money, and would allow me to coach and have adventures at the same time. During my last few weeks living in London I got an email from a team in Poland that was looking for a new head coach for their men's team. After a few emails back and forth the team flew me to Poland for a 24-hour interview. They showed me around the stadium, the city, and introduced me to a lot of big named people in the city. After being wined and dined, I flew back to London feeling confident I had put my best foot forward. One week later they called me to offer me the job of head coach of their men's professional team. It was a dream come true, I was back.

4. CIRCLING BIRDS

I was on top of the world. I had taken eight months to regain control over my life. I was off the anti-depressants, I was healthy and I had landed a dream job. Poland wasn't necessarily on the top of my list of countries to coach in, but it was a stepping-stone and I was happy to have the opportunity. I took a few weeks back home where I was proud to tell people about my new job. I had taken a quantum leap in my career, and more so I felt I had taken a quantum leap and kicked depression out of my life. I was stronger than those anti-depressants. I could out-smart my struggles.

I moved to Poland and quickly settled into my coaching job. Everyday I would be at the stadium preparing the team and trying to bring my values and ideas to the club. I went there with hundreds of ideas that I wanted to apply to the club and team, and I knew that if I could even apply fifty percent of them I'd be doing okay. Turns out I was able to apply none of my ideas.

After a couple months in Poland things started to go to hell. I started to notice behavior from the club manager that I didn't particularly agree with. It went against my philosophy as a coach, leader, and person. He would spend team money on things that were unimportant, and then when it came time to pay my salary and the player's salaries, he would say the team doesn't have any money. He would trash me to the media, saying that I was making terrible coaching decisions, or that I would have the wrong players in the game during key moments of the match. He started to reinstate players that I had released from the team, and to undermine my authority within the team. He was abusive to the players, verbally assaulting them. All in all he was a bad manager and a bully of a person. He fell about forty-five days behind on paying my salary. I set a meeting with him and I told him that he had fifteen days to bring my salary completely up to date or I was going to resign. I wasn't a volunteer, and I wanted him to know that I didn't approve of the way he was running the club.

I wasn't sure if I would actually resign. My team was performing well. We were in first place in our league and on course to win a championship. For my career it would be great to take this losing team, revamp the line-up and then win a championship. It would surely lead to offers from other countries. But at the same time, I was trying to instill values of leadership, honesty and respect into my players. All while I was being asked to turn a blind eye when my management did the opposite. I think the club manager thought he could call my bluff and that I wouldn't actually resign while we were in first place. He knew that he had saved my career and that it would look terrible to resign from a head-coaching job mid-season. No other teams would take me at this point in the season. Day sixty came and went and my salary was still just a bunch of excuses. I frantically made phone calls to advisors and people in the industry that I respected. None of them could offer me any sort of leads on jobs. If I were going to go through with my resignation it would mean having to return home with no job prospects. I agonized about the decision.

In the end my conscience won out. I think I always knew what the right decision was to make but it was a difficult one. I decided that I couldn't stand by and let this guy bully me or my players. If I didn't take action then I was no better than he was. I was not a volunteer and I wasn't about to go back to a unhealthy work situation that had nearly wrecked me. The next day I made an appointment to see him and handed in my written resignation. The manager was shocked. We argued back and forth for a little while but I held my ground. He had his chance to make things right and he wasted it. A few days later I was on a flight back home. I sat on the plane thinking about what I had just done. While part of me knew it was the right decision, the other part of me knew I was heading home, to hopelessness. The depression birds began to circle.

5. I AM WHO I AM

At this point in my life I hadn't lived in my hometown for over a decade, and with nowhere else to go, I was forced to return to it. The depression birds that were circling nested in my head and heart. I came home to an unknown future, with no friends, and my tail between my legs. Was this the end of a job or the end of a career? Could I rebound from this? Depression sank in heavily.

For days on end I wouldn't leave my room. I had no reason to get out of bed. The line from the film *Sleepless in Seattle* played in my head; "If I just put my feet on the floor, and keep breathing, I'll be okay." But it felt so hard to do just that. It felt like so much effort to put my feet on the floor. If I did then I knew I'd have to do something. I'd have to go out into the town and face people that might recognize me. I'd have to look for a job. And finding a job in my hometown would make it official that I had failed and I was here to stay. Out of anger I hired a lawyer in Poland to sue the team for the back-funds they owed me. It was the only thing I could do to try and feel better. I felt if a court would decide in my favor it would prove that I was right to leave.

Things seemed to multiply themselves as I began to realize that not only had I lost my job, but I had been foolish to think that I could "beat" my depression. I began to fear that I was not strong enough. For a long time I had thought that feeling sad was a weakness and if I just concentrated hard enough I'd be able to not feel sad anymore. I believed if I'd just walk around with a smile on my face, despite the fact that inside I was falling apart, that eventually I'd actually feel happy. I began to wonder if I could make it through these dark days.

This terrible feeling lasted for a few months. If I was in town and ran into someone I knew and they asked why I was home I would just say "oh I'm just visiting for Christmas." or "oh my contract is over and now I'm just hanging out." I felt ashamed to be there. And each time I would lie about it I would feel even more depressed.

Eventually I came to a crossroads, I knew I couldn't stay in my room forever, and I needed to either get on with it or give up. My stubborn head told me that I'm not giving up and that I'm going to just get on with it. I slowly started to get out of the house. I took a job, then a second job, and even a third job. I started to go to the gym and to meet some new friends. From the time I got home it had taken me about six months to get through this dark place and get back onto my feet. It was one of the hardest times of my life.

One day I was watching TV and a show came on about depression. It was a documentary by Michael Landsberg called *Darkness and Hope* about athletes who suffer from depression. Being something that I was still ashamed of and still hid, it was really moving for me to see these sports people talk about their struggles. It was like the documentary was written just for me. It was people in my own field that were admitting the same struggles I had. They were saying to me "hey, I've been where you are." Suddenly it wasn't such a lonely place. In the coming week I watched and re-watched the documentary about a dozen times. It gave me courage to talk about depression and it gave me courage to share how I was feeling with people. ***That changed everything for me.***

Suddenly people began to hear me talk about depression and maybe motivated by my openness, felt they could confide in me. I had no idea it was all around me. Friends and people I had known all my life came out of the woodwork and started to tell me about their struggle with depression. I was shocked and comforted that I wasn't alone. I realized that one of the most helpful things for me, especially on dark days, was to tell someone. For years I had been hiding how I felt. Thinking I shouldn't bother other people, or they wouldn't understand. Thinking that it would make me sound weak or lame. But I realized that if I knew other people who were in the same boat as me, and they could relate to my feelings, that it would help me. Just like when they came to talk to me in their dark days that it helped them. To this day, anytime I speak to a group and share about my struggle with depression, there is *always* someone who comes up to me to say they struggle too, and to thank me for talking about it.

Slowly my realization and relationship with depression changed. It started as something I was ashamed of, that I tried to hide away from friends and family. Then it became something I needed to conquer or beat. I felt like I was a smart person and if I could just focus all my brainpower I could out-smart this illness. Then when I came back from Poland and the illness reared it's ugly head, I realized the power it had over me. And my relationship changed again, now I realized that depression wasn't something that I beat or out-smart. It was a part of me. It was a part of who I was and how I was put together. Just like my hair color or my height, it's a part of my make up. Rather than try to cure myself from the illness, I needed to just accept it. This is me, this is a part of who I am, now lets just get on with it. It wasn't drugs or therapy that changed things for me. It was just accepting my illness, being open to talk about it, and being willing to share with people when I needed help. I am who I am.

6. MILE SEVENTEEN

In reflecting back on my interactions with depression, I realize that part of my problems were due to the things going on inside my body - but part of the problems were also how I was living my life. I am an ambitious guy. I like to be busy. In some ways I became afraid of being bored. When boredom set in then I would be left to reflect on my feelings and myself. That can be a scary place when you can't control your feelings.

A few years ago I took on the challenge to complete a full marathon. I'm not in incredible shape and I'm by no means a long distance runner. But I set the goal to complete the marathon and I started training. As the day of the marathon approached, people would ask if I was nervous or ready for it, questions that I didn't really know how to answer. By the 5th mile all the excitement of the starting line had faded and now you were on your own. By the 10th mile you were in your groove and feeling good. At the 17-mile mark I reached my discovery point. In my training, partly due to fear, and partly due to injury, I never did a training run that was longer than 17 miles. So when I passed that 17-mile marker I knew I was in uncharted territory for my body, and my mind. By mile 21 I was thinking how stupid marathons are, why would someone ever want to do this? By mile 23 I knew that no injury or force of nature could stop me from finishing, I'd come that far, I wasn't going to stop now. Then the finish line came and I had done it. In just under five hours I had completed the entire full marathon – 26 miles. It felt great to accomplish the goal. My body felt physically tired and sore on a cellular level. It was like each individual cell that makes up the muscle was sore and tired. But when people would ask what the hardest part was, I'd tell them that spending five hours in my head was pretty tough. When you run, you get into this rhythm or zone and after a while everything else around you fades away. You just fall into your mind and your body automatically keeps putting one foot in front of the other. Spending five hours in my own mind, any other time would terrify me. But I had accomplished it. I had survived.

In my life I wasn't putting myself first. I thought that it was being "humble" to put everyone else's needs ahead of my own. I thought it was making myself a "humble hard worker" to put in 60 hour weeks when it didn't change my salary. It wasn't being humble. It was being stupid. When I moved to London to recharge my batteries I realized that I needed to take time to do things that I enjoyed. I was sitting at a coffee shop one afternoon and saw a flyer for "Adult Kung Fu Lessons". I thought it sounded cool so I signed up. It became something I looked forward to every week. I'm by no means a martial arts expert but I enjoyed doing something for me. To take time out of my life to do something I enjoyed. It was one of the first times that I was doing something that didn't have to do with my career. It helped me realize that my life didn't need to revolve around my work. That I could still be great at my job even if I took time off, went on holidays, or enjoyed other activities. I realized that in order to be humble in my life and my work, I needed to first take care of myself. *My job description wasn't my self-description.* I also learned that "no" is a complete sentence - and I didn't have to agree with or accept everything that was asked of me and my time. People always wanted me to help them, or cover a shift, or do something for them, and it would just eat up all my time. Now days I say "no" more than I say yes. Not because I'm selfish, but because of the value of my free time. I know that if I open the door to letting someone else control my life or my time, that it's a hard door to close.

Today I've discovered a few things that have helped me open up, enjoy spending time "in my head", and give me hope.

7. SMALL STORIES

When I was young I used to write short stories. They would be little stories about things that were happening around me. I tried to model the stories after the great Stuart MacLean's *Vinyl Cafe* stories. When I was about 15-16 years old I wrote a collection of stories that I felt were a good depiction of my childhood and life at the time. Then my "adult" life started and the stories lay dormant on my hard drive collecting computer dust in a folder somewhere. I never forgot about the stories, I always made sure that whenever I was transferring to a new computer, that the stories came with me, but I never did anything with them.

Fast forward to 2011. I was coming out of my dark depression after Poland and I was looking for a project that I could focus on. Something that I would be passionate about, that would give me some energy to work on each day. A reason to get out of bed. I decided to take a look at those old stories. I went onto my computer and printed them all off and then started to read them. A couple of the stories made me laugh, some brought tears to my eyes, and others made me cringe. But through all of them I kept feeling there was something to work with. So I started to re-write the stories. I went through and fixed up the grammar, spelling, and flow. I wrote a couple new stories to beef up the collection a bit and then I started to research publishing. I found a self-publishing company and submitted my manuscript. They sent it to an editor who hacked and whacked it and then sent me back a dozen or so stories to put together into a book. In May 2012 I got the first copy of *Small Stories* from the printer. I was so thrilled to have an actual book in my hands. Wow, what a great feeling. It was amazing to be able to show my friends and family this book that I had published. Then a couple of small bookstores started to stock my book and it started to sell on Amazon. It was a really exciting project.

Small Stories is not the greatest book ever written, but it's a fun, simple read that will bring people back to their childhood. But more importantly it was a turning point in my life. When I had this project it gave me something to focus my life around. I wasn't thinking about my illness anymore. I was excited about this new adventure I was going on. To this day *Small Stories* has a special place in my heart because it was an accomplishment, a goal, something that gave me hope. Like the jacket from my first traveling hockey team, or the jersey from my junior hockey team, or the medal for completing the full marathon, this book was a memento that I could do what I set my mind too. In the moments that I was writing, I wasn't thinking about Poland or my career. I wasn't thinking about being sad or angry, I was just taken away to these fun stories from my childhood. Having this project slowly gave me the courage to step out of my room and my house.

My second book, *The Wandering Leader* is the book I was meant to write, I felt called to write that book. *The Wandering Leader* is a book about leadership and personal development. In it I share a lot of personal experiences and stories about over-coming obstacles, including depression, to be a successful leader. I had to start my writing with fiction though. *Small Stories*, although based on real experiences from my own life, are fictional stories. At the time in my life I wasn't at a healthy enough place mentally or emotionally to write non-fiction. So writing fiction helped me slowly heal myself and get back to a healthy place.

Today my writing is an important part of my life. It helps me organize my thoughts and feelings. I have exciting ideas for two or three more books. I don't know if I'm a good writer and personally I don't really care. The writing helps me feel comfortable spending time in my own head. And the books that come out of the writing I call *Hope Projects*.

8. THE HOPE PROJECT

Hope Projects are something that I now need in my life. It is something that I can focus on, that I'm passionate about and that give me hope. They give me hope that I can accomplish things I set my mind too, that I have some talent, and that I can help other people. These three things are important when setting up a Hope Project.

I want to encourage everyone, especially those who struggle with depression, to start a Hope Project. It can be anything. I started with something that I enjoyed doing, writing. That is the first ingredient in having a Hope Project. Enjoy it. There is no point in making a Hope Project doing something that you don't like. If your project is to build custom furniture, but you hate working with wood and tools, then it's probably not a good choice. Pick something you enjoy doing or something you've always wanted to do. On those days where dark cloud have you sopped in, your enjoyment of the task is what will get you out of bed or out of the house. The fun and love of the project is what will give you that ounce of motivation to leave your darkness.

Your project can be anything, but it shouldn't be for your boss or work. It should be something that gives your mind total freedom from the day to day. For me it was to write and publish a book. I never thought that I would be able to replace my income with book sales, I dreamed it, but I never thought it would actually happen. It's okay to dream things like that. It's okay to dream that maybe your book will go viral, that it will be flying off the shelves and that you'll skyrocket up the New York Times bestseller list. It's exciting to have that dream. The dream, although maybe it's not realistic, gives you excitement and energy. Energy that is important when doing the smallest things in daily life seem to use all your energy up. The Anglo-Saxon word for "happiness" comes from the root word that means, "dream". So dreaming creates happiness. Allow yourself to dream.

I visited Auschwitz Concentration Camp while I was in Poland. I wanted to go through the tour of the camp and find a lesson I could teach with. I couldn't do it. I ended up having a difficult time finding any lesson from the tour. In a place where they considered suicide to be a luxury, there was no hope. I started to wonder then, what was the lesson? What could we learn from visiting a place like that? The best thing I could come up with was dreaming. The only thing that the prisoners had was their dreams. Dreams of life, of food, of family, of freedom. Dreams that would allow them to escape their reality, if even for a few brief minutes. Allow yourself to dream.

The second part of having a Hope Project is to do something that you have some talent in, or want to further develop talent in. English was always a strong subject for me so writing came naturally. I'm an introverted person so writing was a way for me to express myself to others through words. I felt that maybe I had some sort of talent in writing so it was worth exploring. I wasn't starting from scratch. Since my first book was published and I've really started writing on a daily basis, my writing has changed and improved, and hopefully it will continue that way for the rest of my life. I now read books about writing and I identify great writing when I read it. I pick up on things that other writers are doing that I like. But I started with a feeling that I had some talent and that I could possibly do it.

If I were choosing painting pictures as my Hope Project I would soon quit. Yes, I could take a class in painting and maybe learn some of the skills involved in painting, but I know I have no artistic abilities and I know that I would get discouraged. Even if I was taking a class or a course to learn it, I would have many small failures early on, and these would be discouraging. A Hope Project needs to excite us. It needs to give us something to look forward to every day. By choosing a topic that you feel you've already got some talent or skill in it gives you some small victories early on. These small victories help to encourage your Hope Project. For me it would be in completing a story for my book. Each time I would finish a story and reread it, it would be a small victory for me. Then it was getting that first draft of my bound book. Seeing that draft of the manuscript in book form, even though it still had mistakes, gave me a small victory. It gave me motivation to continue with my project, and to work through those mistakes. If I was taking an art class, and my first assignment was to paint a simple picture, I know I would get so frustrated with it that I would give up. I have no talent at painting or drawing. So choose your first Hope Project carefully. I'm not saying don't learn new things, but don't make those new things your Hope Project until you feel like you've got a bit of skill in it.

The final part of the Hope Project is that it should help someone else. It doesn't have to change someone's life. But it just needs to help enrich someone's life a bit. My book *Small Stories* was an easy read, simple stories, and brought people back to their own childhoods. It helped them remember things that they did when they were young and it made them laugh. That feeling of enriching other people's lives is the reward. Making $1.00 on a book sale is not the reward. But getting an email from a reader who says that one moment of the stories made them laugh, or brought back memories of their own childhood is what makes it worthwhile. No matter what you choose, from knitting mittens, to making wood furniture, to painting pictures. It needs to make someone's life brighter. I have a friend who does airbrushing on cars and people's toys (snowboards, helmets, fridges, etc..) He is really talented and he loves to do it. I asked him if he would paint something for me, and he came up with the most beautiful design. The colors are bright and the images jump out at you almost like they're 3D. He painted a beautiful water picture with a Koi fish swimming and a reflection of a face in the ripples of the water. It's truly amazing. This little painting brings me happiness every time I look at it. It speaks peace to me. No matter what you choose as a Hope Project, it should somehow enrich someone else's life. The funny thing is that when you focus your Hope Project on other people, it will change your life too.

9. THE GAME CHANGER

After I had gotten into the writing scene and writing became a part of my regular daily life, I began to look for a new Hope Project. I wanted to find a Hope Project that would be on a bigger scale - that would change people's lives, and change my life. Enter: Me+

Me+ (pronounced: Me Plus) is a product that I created that was one of my Hope Projects. In early 2012, around the same time I was launching *Small Stories*, I started a company called Small World Inc. The company was a website where I could take all my little muses and interests and put them into one place. One of the sub-companies was called Small World Health. Small World Health was originally a platform that I could use to promote health products that I was using or thought were good. There were some great products there, products for weight loss, or vitamins, and even sports nutrition products. They were all great products and I was happy to endorse them for other companies. But I wanted something of my own. No matter how nice it was to promote someone else's product, at the end of the day, it was their win, not my win. I wanted my own wins.

So I started to do research. At the same time that I was researching how to start a nutrition product, I was also looking for a nutrition product that would help me with my feelings of depression. I didn't like being on anti-depressants, and since I went off them while living in England, I didn't want to go back on them. I wanted to find something that would help me steady my feelings. I was buying generic vitamin D and fish oils to help, but it wasn't what I was after.

Part of launching a product is to have a market, and then to niche down in that market. So, if your selling knitted socks, then your market is clothing and your niche market is hand-made customized socks. So while I knew I wanted to be in the vitamin/supplement industry I didn't know how to niche down my product. I was spending a lot of time researching sports supplements but that market is so watered down. There is so much competition there. I also thought about "greens", but again, lots of competition. I can't bring a "Vitamin C" product to the market and think it's going to sell when you can buy Vitamin C in any grocery store in the country. I needed to figure out what my niche market was.

In one of those "ahah" moments, I realized the answer was right in front of me. While I was spending hours researching the supplement market, in my personal life I was trying to find a supplement that didn't exist. I needed to create that depression supplement that *I wanted to buy*. My market was vitamins/supplements and my niche market would be all-natural depression and anxiety supplements. As soon as I had the thought, I knew it was going to work. More importantly, rather than just creating a generic supplement like a protein powder for athletes, I was creating a supplement that I wanted to use myself.

In looking back on the decision to go into the depression market, I think I was afraid to think about that market because I had a feeling I'd have to share my story. In order for the product to really be successful, it has to be personal. I can't just sell another depression supplement, it needs to be personal, it needs to be real. It needs to be born out of a need. This became my new Hope Project, one that I didn't realize would change my life.

10. THE BLUE PRINT

The process of building a proper health supplement is a complicated one; it takes a lot of money and a lot of planning. I learned a lot through the process and I made a lot of mistakes through the process but I was so thrilled the day that Me+ officially launched.

To start building the product I began my listing all of my symptoms that I wanted a product to help me with. First and foremost I wanted a product that would address the imbalances that cause depression. I wanted to have a bit more in control over those feelings. That part of the supplement was obvious, but not good enough, I wanted more. I also wanted more energy. When I was in one of the darkest periods in my life I didn't want to get out of bed. I'm generally a really active person but during those days it felt like my energy was gone. I had no energy to do anything and I'd lie in bed watching Seinfeld reruns. I'd then feel even worse because I'd eat crap, accomplish nothing, and then kick myself for it. So I wanted my new supplement to give me more energy. I wanted something that if I took it, I would have so much energy I'd have no choice to get out of bed and do something. The final thing I wanted was health and mobility. Anti-Depressants can be really harsh on your body. They can break down your kidneys and liver, they come with side effects, and for some people can cause more problems then they help. I wanted my supplement to do the opposite. I wanted my supplement to give me energy and fight depression, but I also wanted it to heal my body. I wanted some kick-ass vitamins and antioxidants in there.

All of these types of products are already available on the Internet. I began to look at who my competition would be. There are some great companies out there, with great products, but nothing that was as much of a total package as what I wanted to build. You could buy all-natural supplements that fight depression. You can buy vitamin and antioxidant supplements to heal your body and joints. You can even buy energy supplements. But at about $25 - $40 each, you'll have to buy three different products, spending over $100 by the time everything is shipped to you. It's too complicated. I didn't want to have to buy three different products, and have three different bottles cluttering up my bathroom, and pay three different bills. I wanted one product that could help me with the things I was struggling with.

I enlisted the help of three doctors to share their knowledge with me. I started to research about different herbs and vitamins. I asked them to research the best ingredients they could think of for my product. I came back with a list of ingredients and submitted it to my manufacturing partner. They ran some tests through their lab to make sure everything was safe and then created a trial of the product.

During the process I came up with the idea for a second product. The first product was a morning product. You'd take it when you wake up, it would give you energy to start your day, give you a good dose of depression help and vitamins. But I also noticed that I struggled to fall asleep. Sometimes I'd lie awake with all sorts of thoughts running through my head. I couldn't shut my brain off. These anxious thoughts would get me wound up and I'd be up for half the night. My morning product would be no good if you can't fall asleep at night. Sleep is where your body recharges, where it heals, where it produces hormones. So I wanted to create a product that would go hand in hand with my morning product. I wanted a product that I could take before bed that would help me shut my brain off and fall asleep.

Finally I got the trial products and was excited to give them a try. Results? Not great. The morning supplement was okay, but not overly noticeable. It wasn't strong enough. The evening supplement was the opposite. It would literally knock you out in about 30 minutes, but then you'd wake up with lots of energy around 3:00 or 4:00am. That's not exactly what I wanted. Back to the drawing board.

Round two of the supplement came about three months later. After going back to meetings with my doctors and with the nutrition lab, we figured out the problems. We tweaked our ingredients and then began to test the second round. Our problem with the sleep supplements was gone but now it wasn't quite strong enough. The morning supplement was better, but still not quite there. I wanted it to be perfect. Yes, the product at this point was probably good enough to go to market with, and I know people benefited from it because some of the friends and family that helped me test it, loved it. But I wanted more. I wanted it to change people's lives. So back to the drawing board we went.

Another three months went by with countless hours researching ingredients and combinations, before the final blend was sent to me for trials. Before I begin to test a new supplement I stop taking all other vitamins and supplements for two weeks before I start the new trial. That way I get a clear idea if I notice any feeling changes. After the first time I took this blend, I knew we had a winner. The morning supplement (Me+ AM "Rise and Shine") gave me an energy boost that I could notice, but didn't make me feel jittery. I had energy that lasted throughout the day and helped me get going in the morning. More so, by adding some amino acids, it also started to help me focus more. The bigger surprise came with the evening supplement (Me+ PM "Sleeping Beauty"). While this was created almost as an after-thought, to me it has become my favorite of the two. I didn't want something that would knock you out. I wanted something that if I took the supplement, and something came up and I had to drive my car, that I wouldn't fall asleep at the wheel. This new blend of the PM supplement was very gentle. The main thing it did was help to quiet my mind using lemon balm extract. Suddenly all those noisy thoughts were turned down and when that happened I would drift off to sleep naturally. And by adding some extracts from tea and leafy greens, I found I was getting really deep, restful sleeps. I would wake up feeling refreshed and ready to go. It was fantastic.

The vitamin blend that is in both products is gentle and hard working. I wanted something that would help my immune system, keeping me healthy. In a recommendation from my baby-boomer father, I added in Glucosamine, a product that heals your joints and cartilage. It's tough to feel like getting out of bed and doing something if your sick or your joints hurt. So I took care of that. Then, on the recommendation of one of my doctor friends, he had told me to research about ginger, and after hours reading about this little root, I had it included it into the evening blend. Ginger naturally helps balance out the pH levels in your stomach - naturally fighting any feelings of heartburn or indigestion. I was so happy with the products. Not only did I want to share them with the world, but also they were helping me live fully day-to-day.

The Hope Project

11. THE C.H.O.

I have a friend who has had a pretty tough life. Like me, he struggles from depression, and we've often spent time talking about it. He was one friend that was supportive of my Hope Project from day one. He trialed the products, gave me feedback, and now today he promotes the products for me. He was the one who came up with the name of the product line, "Me+". We were laughing and joking one day about the product. Saying how it did everything we had hoped, and a bit more. We were joking that on our product we could run faster, jump higher, rescue cats from trees, and pick up chicks. We joked about how it was like "Me, plus more." As soon as he said it, I knew that was the name of the product. Me+.

While this product does not do everything and while it does not cure everything, it does work.

To this day I use it every morning and every evening. I love it. I'm so proud of it. The next step with this Hope Project was to share it with other people in hopes that it would enrich their lives. To start off, I gave my friend who helped me with the name a lifetime supply. He has a secret ordering code that he can go onto our company website and order the product for no charge. I didn't owe him anything and he doesn't expect anything from me, but he loves the product, and it helps him be in control in his life - and to me that's worth supporting. While I wish I could give the product away to everyone who suffers from depression, that wouldn't make much sense from a business stand point. I wanted to do something that would change my life and change the lives of people around me. I wanted to be able to take my Hope Project and be able to "quit my day job."

I put the Small World Inc team to work designing a new website for the product and building a shopping cart feature. My retired father offered to help as our "shipping department" during the start up days. So when an order would come in, I would forward him the order and address and he'd pull out the products, go down to the post office and ship them. He loved being able to help me grow my little business and he loved to keep track of my inventory for me. It was a fun little project that he could do in his retirement. As the company grew I'd eventually end up moving all of our shipments to a drop-shipping warehouse and I'd be free to do other fun things with my dad.

Me+ started as a Hope Project. It started as something that I wanted to do to help me and my friends. It has now grown into an international business and through the money that I earn from product sales I'm able to research new products, but more importantly (and more fun) I can come up with ways to help others. We want to develop a scholarship fund. We want to run contests with our loyal customers. We've hired a CHO (Customer Happiness Officer) whose job it is to contact customers and make sure they're happy with the product and service. The CHO has a "Random Acts of Kindness" budget that he can use each month to make people's day. He can give away our product or he can go and buy something online for a customer and just surprise them. We want to brighten people's days because we know what it's like to fight the battles against depression. (Last month our CHO bought theatre tickets for one customer living in New York City - the customer was so thrilled to be able to go spend a night out at the theatre with her husband that she called our Customer

Care line and left a very emotional voicemail message. Messages like that give me hope that I'm doing the right thing.)

Now my new Hope Projects are ways I can make people smile. One day I'd like to be able to build a house for myself and start a family. One day I'd like that dream house on the backside of the family island and make homemade wine from the grapes I'll plant. One day I'd like to have a an education fund for my God-kids. But for today, I want to help other people by sharing my story. Today I really want to be Me+.

12. START SMALL

The Hope Project for me has changed my life and my view on life. When I was waging war on depression it seemed my life was total chaos. But once I began having a Hope Project it gave me new focus and new control over my life. You need to start your Hope Project today. It doesn't need to replace your income, it doesn't even need to provide income at all, it just needs to be a project that you can focus on to give you hope. My Hope Project started very simple, just writing a few stories. Keep your Hope Project simple.

I believe that everyone has a book in them. Maybe you can make it your Hope Project to write a book. It's takes some work but you can write a book, self-publish it and share it with family and friends. You'll be amazed at the feeling to hold your own book in your hand. Even something like creating a photo album through iPhoto or another app is rewarding. Maybe you want to start a small company selling something you can make. Use the model I outlined with the Me+ product. It doesn't have to be a vitamin, it can be anything, cookies, bread, scarves, hats, wooden pens, vases, socks, whatever you're good at, make it, share it.

A couple final pointers about Hope Projects. Don't go into debt with your Hope Project. Personally I don't believe in debt. One of the biggest causes of stress in people's lives is problems with money. So if you've put a bunch of money into your Hope Project, it is going to stress you out and that's not what we want. My Hope Project started as my writing. Then I made the decision that the money I made from *Small Stories* would be put towards funding the creation of Me+. (Today 100% of the sales from *Small Stories* goes to Kids Help Phone.) Some books on building businesses will tell you to go max out a credit card because then you'll feel obligated to succeed. Don't do that. Go slow, let your project take a few months, or even years. But invest yourself in it. For me it was coming to grips with my story. Learning to not be ashamed of my illness and to learn how to talk about it. It's not easy sharing about something that can be perceived as a weakness, but I know that whenever I do it helps other people.

Start small and let your Hope Project grow on it's own. Lets say your idea is making custom wooden picture frames. Do your first few frames as gifts for people that you love. When you make something for someone you love, part of that love is in the product. Other people can see that. I love myself and my friends who suffer from depression, and when I was making Me+ I had them in mind. I believe that love for them made my product better. As word spreads about your custom wooden picture frames you can figure out how you're going to grow it into a small business or project, but don't worry about that in the beginning.

Give back. Part of a Hope Project is that it has to enrich someone else's life. But if your hope project starts to turn into a small business, like Me+, then you need to give back. Support people, charities, and ideas that you believe in. Support things that make the world a better place. You don't need to give back financially, but you can support people and businesses with your time, your love and your knowledge. Share your story. Listen to their stories. We're part of a bigger community and when we realize that it helps to make the days a bit brighter.

Reach out. Ask for help when you get stuck. I didn't know the legal requirements for starting a vitamin supplement, so I reached out to a friend who was a lawyer who could help me. I didn't know how to set up an online store, so I sought out people to help me and advise me in my business. But more important, not every day is a perfect day for me, and I've learned that I need to reach out when I'm down. I need to be more open and honest with how I'm feeling. Good and bad. Happy and sad. Don't go through it alone.

13 TAKE A STEP

I have a business friend who has a motto that says "I'm 100% focused on happiness." What a great motto. What happens if we focus all our energy on being happy? If we focus our whole lives to getting better and being happy? For me it was deciding I want to live like a "Rock Star". I'm going to do what I want, when I want, how I want, as long as it makes me happy. Happiness is all that matters for me. My business, my writing, my family and friends all make me happy, so I'm going to keep doing those things.

I want to encourage you that you're not alone in your journey to happiness. Take action today. If there is a product out there that will help you be happy then I believe that your happiness and your health is worth every penny. Take action today. Don't wait for someone else to make you happy, it will never happen. You'll be waiting for a long time. Make the decision today that you're going to be happy. You're not going to accept being sad anymore. Yes, sad days will come and go, but they will no longer be in control. Take your life back. Try creating your own Hope Project by take our 90-day challenge. Here's how it works.

90-Day Hope Project Challenge

Step 1) Write down your Hope Project (set a goal). Remember it should be something that you feel you have some talent it and enjoy doing and will brighten someone else's life. Allow yourself to dream.

Step 2) Write down a few steps to achieve your Hope Project - one of those steps you should be able to complete TODAY and one you should be able to achieve by the end of the week. Get started now, and try to give yourself a few small victories early on.

Step 3) Give yourself 90 days to really get into your Hope Project. Spend a little bit of time on it each week. Try to make a routine around it. Remember it needs to enrich someone else's life too, so be ready to share it. Anytime the depression birds are circling, try spending time working on your Hope Project.

Step 4) Let us know how it went. Share your story with our community.

If after 90 days of trying you don't feel any different in your life, then you can quit. Write me an email (dave@smallworldinc.net) and tell me it didn't work. But, I have a sneaking suspicion that you'll enjoy having a project in your life. If you follow the steps of the Hope Project then I'm sure you'll feel good. And if after 90 days you don't feel different then you'll of occupied your mind, practiced a skill, and shared something with someone else all for nothing. Not a total waste of time I guess.

If you want to ask some questions along the way, get in touch with me and my Small World staff, we're here to help you. Tell us you read The Hope Project and you have some questions about business or Hope Projects, and we'll get back to you and help you at whatever step you're at in the process. The goal is not to cure depression. The goal is to feel comfortable in our own skill, and help other people realize their potential. The goal is to be there for someone, and to make someone smile. The goal is Hope.

AFTERWORD AND BONUSES

I want to get this book into as many people's hands as possible. I want to encourage you that you're not walking alone. While I do have costs associated with printed copies of this book, the eBook is free. I've tried to price the paperback copy as cheap as possible if you want a physical copy.

I need your help now. Share this book with someone you know. I think for most of us we know someone who suffers from depression or anxiety issues and this book might help them. Or share it with your family or friends, so they can get an idea of the things you're struggling with.

I need to share a few quick warnings and disclaimers about Me+. While I spent a lot of time talking about Me+ as an example of building a muse or Hope Project, I am required by law to point out a few little things. First, Me+ products are not meant to cure, treat or prevent depression, anxiety or any other illnesses. Because they have "all-natural" ingredients they are classified as a Food Supplement, and therefore they don't need to be reviewed or approved by the FDA. While we go above and beyond to make sure our products are safe and healthy, we want to make sure people check with their doctors before changing any medications or supplements. We also want people to read all the warnings on the product pages of our website before using Me+. We want you to be safe and happy, so just be smart about it.

If there is anything in this book that you could relate too then we'd love to hear from you. You can email us. You can follow me personally on Twitter, or you can follow Small World Health on Twitter. Post feedback on Amazon or other bookseller sites about this book to help us share our story. We would love if you could help us spread the word about Me+ and this eBook. Join the conversation on Facebook. The more people we reach the more we'll be able to keep helping enrich people's lives and break the silence around depression. You could make it a Hope Project to join our Street Team for the Small World Network if you're talented at promotions and planning, we'd love to welcome you to our team.

If you're struggling with this illness, reach out to someone, and if you feel like you don't have anyone, then reach out to us. We're not professional counselors, but we'll at least listen to you, and sometimes that is enough. We dedicate part of our customer care team specifically to responding to emails from people who are suffering from depression. We're not going to try to sell you something, we're just going to listen.

Finally, for supporting this book we'd like to thank you by giving you some free bonuses. I'd personally like to hear from you and hear your comments on this little handbook. I'd like to give you a free trial of Me+ if you want to try it out, and I'd like to just send you some encouragement that you're not alone in the struggle.

ALSO BY DAVID SMALL

Small Stories

The Wandering Leader

The Wandering Beloved

Blog: www.wanderingleader.com

Me+ is available at www.smallworldhealth.net

ABOUT THE AUTHOR

David Small is a professional ice hockey coach, author and public speaker. David is from Kenora, Ontario Canada and currently travels around the world coaching ice hockey and speaking on leadership. David's first published book *Small Stories* is a collection of fiction short-stories about childhood and supports Kids Help Phone foundation with 100% of the profits. His second book, *The Wandering Leader* is a non-fiction book on leadership and personal development with a theme for athletes. *The Wandering Beloved* carries on David's stories and lessons from *The Wandering Leader* but with a focus on religion.

Take Back Your Happiness Today!

Me+ AM Rise and Shine is going to help you take back your happiness, your energy, and your health. Made with 100% natural ingredients Me+ AM will help you fight feelings of depression, boost your energy, and provides antioxidants and vitamins for overall health. Your health is worth every penny.

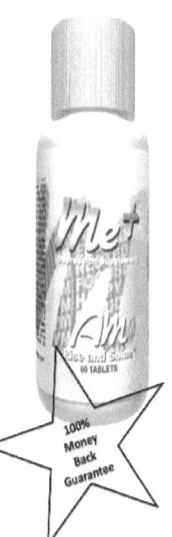

Visit www.smallworldhealth.net to order today!